What Every Nurse Must See Before a Code: Telemetry Secrets

Kristina Michelle, BSN, RN

Dedication

To every nurse-whether you are a student just learning the rhythm of a heart, a new graduate finding your footing, or a seasoned professional with years of experience etched into your hands and heart this book is for you.

It is for the long nights, the quick decisions, the quiet prayers, and the unwavering commitment to your patients. May these pages remind you of the power you hold, the difference you make, and the courage it takes to stand ready in the moments before a code.

You are the heartbeat of healthcare.

Acknowledgment

First and always, I thank God. Every step of this journey has been guided by His hand. In moments of doubt, He gave me clarity. In moments of exhaustion, He gave me strength. And in moments of uncertainty, He reminded me that this path was never meant to be walked alone.

To my family - you have been my safe place and my reason to keep pushing forward. Thank you for your patience, for your understanding when my focus was pulled elsewhere, and for loving me through it all. Your faith in me has been my fuel.

To my mentors you are the voices that have echoed in my heart and mind, urging me to think bigger, dig deeper, and never settle for "good enough." You've shown me the courage it takes to carve out your own way, even when it's not the well-traveled road. Your guidance and belief in me have left an indelible mark on my life.

This book is not just words on a page it's a collection of lessons, prayers, encouragement, and lived experience. And it is for every nurse who stands at the monitor, trusting their training, their instincts, and their heart in the moments before a code.

Contents

Introduction:
Why This Book Matters

What the Monitor Won't Tell You—But You Need to Know

You know that feeling.

You glance up at the telemetry monitor. The rhythm looks... okay. The patient seems fine. But something just doesn't feel right.

And then, hours later, everything changes.

The heart tanks. The labs are off. Someone's running a code. A nurse gets questioned. A chart gets reviewed. And suddenly, you're replaying every moment, every number, every note, wondering what could've been done differently.

I've been there.

Here's the truth no one told you in nursing school:

Rhythms don't kill people. Patterns do.

It's not just the strip— it's the *labs, the vitals, the story.*

Nursing today isn't about memorizing textbook definitions of rhythms. It's about critical thinking. Clinical judgment. Knowing when to worry— and when to act. But the reality is, many nurses were never really taught how to **connect the dots** between what they see on the monitor and what's happening in the body.

We were trained to:

- Identify a rhythm
- Call the provider
- Chart what we were told

But we weren't always taught:

- Why do certain labs affect the strip
- What a U-wave is really telling you
- How replacing potassium without checking magnesium can trigger torsades
- When a "normal" rhythm is lying to you
- Or how documentation could be the only thing standing between you and a board complaint

That's where this book comes in.

This isn't a dry telemetry manual. It's a **real-world guide**— built for nurses who work on telemetry floors, stepdown units, med-surg with monitors, ICUs, and EDs. It's for new grads who want to feel confident interpreting rhythms. It's for seasoned nurses who've trusted their gut and been right. And it's especially for those who want to protect their patients and their license.

Inside, you'll find:

- Straightforward explanations of rhythms without the fluff
- Visuals and case-based lessons that show what real rhythm changes look like
- Lab-to-rhythm connections that help you understand the "why" behind what you're seeing
- Critical thinking tools that go beyond "just call the doc"
- Legal insights that show how charting can help or hurt you
- Personal stories, cheat sheets, escalation tips, and bedside wisdom

Whether you're learning telemetry for the first time or you've been brushing off U-waves for years, I promise you'll learn something here that could make you a safer, smarter, more empowered nurse.

This book won't teach you how to be perfect.

But it *will* help you become the kind of nurse who knows when to speak up, when to push back, and when to trust the pattern your patient is showing you, even if no one else sees it yet.

Let's get into it.

Part 1:

The Heart's Electrical Language

Chapter 1: What the Monitor Isn't Telling You

Telemetry isn't just about beeps. It's about the story behind them.

You walk into your shift. The board lights up with names, bed numbers, and color-coded alerts. Your patient list loads, and the telemetry monitor is already barking at you. Beep. Ding. Atrial fib. Bradycardia. Lead off. PVCs. Lead off again. You silence it.

Sound familiar?

As nurses, we've all been trained to read the monitor, but most of us were never taught to *listen* to it.

I don't mean just identifying a rhythm and checking it off your flowsheet. I'm talking about truly interpreting what it's saying about your patient's physiology, what it could be predicting, and how it connects to their labs, their medications, their overall clinical picture, and yes, your legal risk.

The Illusion of a "Stable" Rhythm

Let's say you're looking at a patient with a normal sinus rhythm at 78 bpm. PR interval's fine. QRS is narrow. QTc looks okay. You chart it: "NSR, no ectopy."

But something feels...off.

The patient's breathing is a little faster. Their BP is dropping. They look pale. The rhythm hasn't changed *yet*.

So, you keep watching. And within hours, they're in V-tach. Or you're pressing the code blue button.

What went wrong?

Nothing on the monitor changed, but *everything else did.*

That's the disconnect this book will help you fix.

Nurses Need Pattern Recognition, Not Just Strip Identification

Telemetry isn't just an academic exercise; it's one piece of a puzzle. The most dangerous mistake we can make is to look at an ECG in isolation. Instead, think of it as a *vital sign with a backstory.*

Here's what I mean:

- A bradycardic strip could be fine, or it could be the **first sign of hyperkalemia.**
- Frequent PVCs might be dismissed, or they might be **hypoxia's SOS before arrest.**

- A prolonged QT interval might go unnoticed until it becomes **torsades.**

These aren't rare, freak incidents. They happen all the time, and I see them in nursing documentation over and over again. One missed lab value. One undocumented call. One silent rhythm change. And suddenly the nurse is on the hook.

You're Not Just a Monitor Watcher - You're a Clinical Interpreter

I can't tell you how many times I've reviewed nursing documentation where the nurse charted "telemetry monitored," but didn't act on a trend, or didn't correlate it with the patient's labs or symptoms. Even though they had all the tools, the telemetry, the vitals, the labs- nobody *put them together.*

Let me be clear: this is not about blaming the nurse. It's about **equipping the nurse.**

Because when no one teaches you how to read between the lines, you're just trying to survive your shift. But if you learn how to recognize patterns— *real patterns*— you become a different kind of nurse: the kind that catches things early, the kind that saves lives, the kind that can back up every decision with sound documentation.

3 Myths About Cardiac Monitoring That Could Cost You Your License

1. "The Tele Tech Will Let Me Know If Something's Wrong."

False.

Monitor techs are a helpful layer, but you are responsible for interpreting telemetry in real-time for your assigned patients. If something goes unnoticed or isn't reported, the legal burden still lands on the licensed nurse. Courts don't care if you "weren't told." They'll ask:

"Did you assess the rhythm yourself?"

Lesson: Always confirm with your own eyes. Never delegate critical thinking.

2. "If the Rhythm Is Sinus, Then the Patient Is Fine."

Dangerously False.

A patient can be in perfect sinus rhythm and still be critically ill, hypoxic, septic, bleeding, and acidotic. The strip is not a full picture. It's one clue. Nurses who ignore subtle changes because "the strip looks normal" often miss decompensation until it's too late.

Lesson: Always correlate the rhythm with vitals, labs, and your physical assessment. A quiet monitor doesn't mean a stable patient.

3. "I Documented It - That's Enough."

Not even close.

Documentation means nothing if you didn't act on what you saw. Did you escalate? Recheck labs? Follow up? Notify the provider with proper urgency? Just noting "telemetry monitored" or "PVCs noted" won't protect you in court if the patient deteriorated and you didn't intervene.

Lesson: Good documentation reflects good nursing actions, not just observations.

Bottom Line:

Telemetry isn't just technology. It's a tool, and you're the clinician who gives it meaning. Don't outsource your judgment. *Own it.*

What This Book Will Teach You (That Nursing School Didn't)

Over the next few chapters, you'll learn:

- How to actually read a rhythm strip and understand what it means
- How to spot dangerous trends even in "normal" rhythms

- What labs correlate with specific rhythm changes, and why
- When to escalate, what to document, and how to protect your license
- Real stories of nursing wins and near-misses, and how you can learn from them

You'll also get charts, checklists, and visual guides that you can use on your next shift, not just in theory, but in practice.

And perhaps most importantly, you'll walk away with the **confidence** to say, "This doesn't look right" and know exactly *why* it doesn't.

Your Role in Patient Safety (and Your Own)

You are the eyes and ears of your patient's heart.

Not the telemetry tech.

Not the doctor who rounds for 90 seconds.

You.

Your assessment, your voice, and your documentation are the first line of defense for your patient *and* your license.

And in the legal world, if it's not documented, it didn't happen. But if it *is* documented, and you didn't act on it? That's just as dangerous.

This book is here to help you do both: make good decisions and show that you made them.

A Quick Story Before We Dive In

Years ago, I had a patient on a step-down unit with sinus tachycardia at 105. New admit. Post-op. Everyone brushed it off- "just pain." But I had that gut feeling.

BP was low-ish. The temp was borderline. He had mild abdominal distension but wasn't complaining. I called the doctor anyway. Got a CT. Perforated bowel. Went to surgery in an hour. Lived.

Was it the rhythm alone that told me that? No.

It was the **pattern**: rhythm + vitals + assessment. That's what saved him.

And that's what this book will help you see.

In the next chapter, I'll break down the anatomy of a rhythm strip in a way that makes sense, even if you haven't looked at telemetry since nursing school..

Then we'll start layering in clinical clues, labs, and real-world judgment.

By the end, you'll know what to look for, what to question, and what to document - because once you know how to truly listen to what the heart is saying, you'll never look at the monitor the same way again.

Chapter 2: Anatomy of a Rhythm Strip - Simplified

Telemetry doesn't have to feel like Greek. The problem is that most nurses were taught to *memorize* rhythms instead of truly *understanding* them. So, let's break it down- not with flashcards, but with common sense.

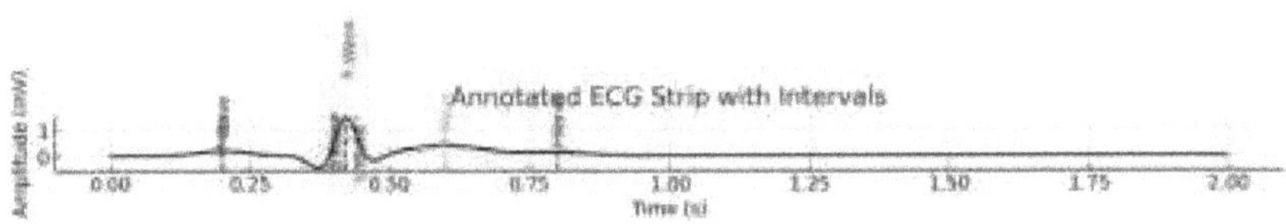

What You're Looking At: The PQRSTU

The ECG waveform is a visual representation of the heart's electrical activity. Each bump, dip, and segment tells a part of the story:

❖ **P Wave**

- **What it is:** Atrial depolarization (when the atria contract)
- **What to look for:** Is it upright? Consistent? Does it always show up before a QRS?
- **Red flags:** Absent or inconsistent P waves could be atrial fibrillation or junctional rhythms

❖ **Q Wave**

- What it is: The first negative deflection after the P wave (beginning of ventricular depolarization)
- What to look for: Small Q waves are normal. Deep or wide Q waves can signal prior MI.
- Red flags: Pathologic Q waves, infarct pattern on 12-lead

❖ **R Wave**

- What it is: The main positive spike of ventricular contraction
- What to look for: Height, spacing, and regularity
- Red flags: Tall R waves in V1-V2RVH; loss of progression, anterior infarct

❖ **S Wave**

- What it is: The downward deflection following the R wave
- What to look for: Completes the QRS complex
- Red flags: Wide QRS (>0.12s) → bundle branch blocks, hyperkalemia, or ventricular rhythms

❖ T Wave

- What it is: Ventricular repolarization (the "reset")
- What to look for: Upright, rounded, not peaked
- Red flags: Tall, peaked T waves indicate hyperkalemia, inverted Ischemia, Flattened T hypokalemia

❖ **U Wave**

- What it is: Late repolarization, often due to hypokalemia or hypomagnesemia
- What to look for: Small bump after the T wave
- Red flags: Prominent U waves + PVCs, electrolyte imbalance that can trigger torsades

Intervals and Durations (And Why They Matter)

Interval	Normal range	What it means
PR interval	0.12-0.20 sec	AV node delay longer than 1st-degree block
QRS duration	< 0.12 sec	Time for ventricles to contract
QT interval	0.44 sec (corrected)	Prolonged risk for torsades, esp. with low Mg/K

Clinical Pearls for the Real World

- Always measure **PR and QT intervals** when rhythms change suddenly.
- Don't ignore **U waves,** they're whispers before chaos (think torsades).
- **P waves without QRS?** You've got a block, look deeper.

- If it's wide, **it's either sick or faking it** (check for artifact or bundle branch block).

Rhythm Isn't Just Electrical - It's Clinical

Imagine a patient in NSR. Looks good, right?

But they're weak, dizzy, and their labs just came back with:

- K: 2.9
- Mg: 1.4
- QTc: 0.52

Suddenly, that "normal" strip isn't so reassuring.

That **U wave** you didn't notice? Now it matters.

That's what this chapter and this book are about:

Learning to see what matters before it becomes a crisis.

Chapter 3: How to Think Like a Cardiac Nurse

Reading rhythms is one thing. Thinking like a cardiac nurse? That's what saves lives.

You know what separates a nurse who reads telemetry from one who interprets it?

Clinical thinking.

It's not about memorizing PQRST sequences. It's about understanding the why behind a rhythm, what labs and signs support it, and whether what you're seeing makes sense with what the patient is doing or not doing.

Telemetry will give you a clue. The patient will give you the story. It's your job to connect them.

A Quick Tour of the Heart's Electrical Highway

Cardiac Conduction System

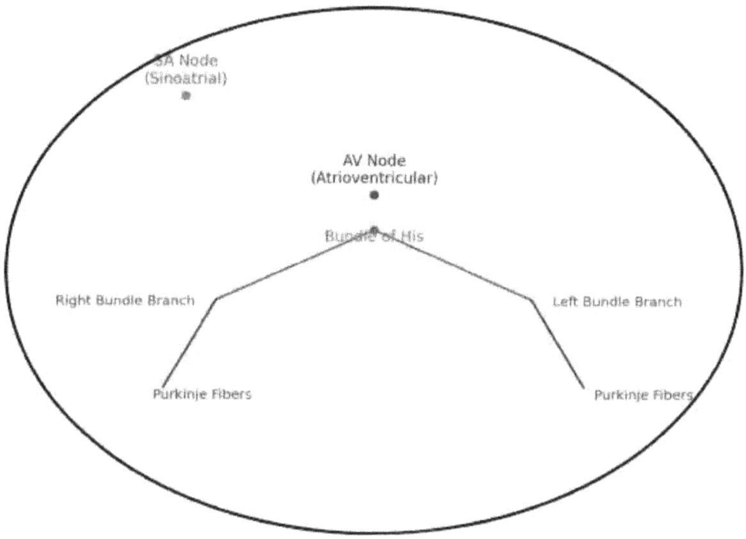

Before we dive deeper, let's go over where all these rhythms come from.

Your telemetry monitor isn't just picking up waves. It's showing the **electrical signal's journey through the heart.** If there's a madblock anywhere, it changes the rhythm and sometimes the outcome

Here's the fast-track version:

❖ **SA Node (Sinoatrial Node)**

- The heart's natural pacemaker is located in the right atrium
- Fires at 60-100 bpm (normal sinus rhythm)

- If it fails, other parts of the heart try to take over, but slower and shakier.

- ❖ **AV Node (Atrioventricular Node)**
  - The gatekeeper between the atria and ventricles
  - Delays the impulse just long enough to let the ventricles fill
  - Fires at 40-60 bpm if the SA node fails
  - Too much delay? That's a **heart block.**

- ❖ **Bundle of His, Bundle Branches, and Purkinje Fibers**
  - This is the "wiring" down the ventricles
  - Conducts the impulse fast to cause a coordinated contraction
  - Right or left bundle branch block? Expect a **wide QRS**
  - If these fail, the ventricles take over at 20-40 bpm, and that's not sustainable

Key concept:

The further down the conduction system the rhythm originates, the slower and more dangerous it tends to be.

You don't need to be a cardiologist to understand this. You just need to know that if the **AV node is holding too long**, or the ventricles are pacing themselves, you'll see it in the **rate, rhythm, and QRS shape.**

This electrical map is what you're seeing on telemetry. Once you understand it, the rhythm makes more sense because you'll know where the problem starts.

Quick Reference: Thinking Like a Cardiac Nurse

Ask Yourself	Why It Matters
Where is this rhythm originating? (SA. AV, ventricles?)	The lower it starts, the slower and riskier it gets
Is this rhythm appropriate for the patient's condition?	Sinus rhythm in a hypotensive or septic patient isn't always reassuring.
Are labs contributing to what I see?	Electrolytes are often the silent culprit.
What am I doing about this?	Assessment without action = risk
Did I document all this clearly?	Protect your license and show your thinking.

Heart Rate, Preload/Afterload, and Perfusion: The Bigger Picture

Now let's tie everything together. When you look at a rhythm, you also need to ask yourself: *Why is the heart behaving this way?* The heart doesn't just beat randomly. Every beat has to be synchronized with the body's demands.

That's where **preload**, **afterload**, and **perfusion** come into play. These factors influence the heart's performance, including the rhythm you see on the monitor. Let's break each one down:

❖ Heart Rate: More Than Just a Number

The heart rate is the most obvious and easy-to-read part of the rhythm strip, but it's also one of the most misunderstood. A "normal" heart rate at rest is 60-100 bpm, but **rate alone doesn't tell you the full story.**

- **Tachycardia** can be a compensatory response to stress, blood loss, or hypoxia.
- **Bradycardia** might reflect a protective response (e.g., vagal tone) or indicate a failure in the conduction system (e.g., heart block).

- You should always ask: Why is this heart rate what it is? Is it compensating for something? Is it inadequate for perfusion?

❖ Preload: The Heart's Filling Pressure

Preload refers to the **amount of blood returning to the heart,** particularly the ventricles, before contraction. It's essentially the **"stretch"** of the heart muscle; more blood means more stretch, which should generate a stronger contraction.

- **High preload** (e.g., in heart failure or fluid overload) increases the workload of the heart, possibly leading to arrhythmias like atrial fibrillation.
- **Low preload** (e.g., hypovolemia, hemorrhage) can reduce cardiac output, leading to tachycardia as the heart tries to compensate.

❖ Afterload: The Heart's Resistance to Ejection

Afterload is the **resistance the heart faces when pumping blood** into the arteries. Higher afterload means the heart must work harder to get the blood out.

- Conditions like **hypertension** or **aortic stenosis** increase afterload, which can contribute to left ventricular hypertrophy, arrhythmias, and a high risk for heart failure.
- **Low afterload** (e.g., from sepsis or vasodilation) can also lead to hypotension and inadequate perfusion, which stresses the heart, especially in low-output states.

❖ Perfusion: The Endgame of Heart Function

Ultimately, **perfusing tissues with oxygenated blood** is the heart's job, and if that's not happening, the heart itself will suffer.

- A patient with **poor perfusion** (e.g., from low BP, shock, or poor heart function) might look stable on telemetry, but their tissues are in distress.
- **Signs of poor perfusion:**
  - Pale, cool skin
  - Low urine output
  - Altered mental status
  - Tachycardia or bradycardia as compensatory responses

Key concept:

When heart rate, preload, and afterload aren't balanced, you'll start seeing the effects on perfusion, and it can show up in the rhythm. If the rhythm looks fine but the patient's perfusion is compromised, don't just rely on the monitor to tell you what's going wrong.

The Cardiac Nurse's Mental Checklist

Ask Yourself	Why it Matters
Where is this rhythm originating? (SA, AV, ventricles?)	The lower it starts, the slower and more dangerous it gets
What's the heart rate telling me? Is it compensating, too fast, or too slow?	Tachycardia can signal compensation; bradycardia can indicate conduction failure.
Is preload, afterload, or perfusion a factor?	High or low preload/afterload affects the heart's ability to pump effectively, leading to arrhythmias.
Are labs contributing to what I see?	Electrolyte imbalances, acidosis, and hypoxia can change the rhythm and worsen perfusion.
Did I document everything clearly?	Good documentation reflects both your assessment and your interventions.

Telemetry doesn't just tell you what the heart is doing. It tells you what the **body** is doing. Your job is to read between the lines and between the beeps.

When you understand **heart rate, preload, afterload,** and **perfusion,** you can think critically about what's really happening. This chapter is about **putting those pieces together.**

In the next chapter, we'll dive into **bradycardias and blocks** and how to tell when "slow" is sleepy, sick, or headed for a crash.

Part 2: When Rhythms Get Real

Chapter 4: Bradycardias and Blocks -When Slow Means Trouble

Not all slow rhythms are stable. Some are trying to tell you the heart is dying.

At first glance, a slow heart rate might not alarm anyone.

Sinus bradycardia? Normal in athletes.

Junctional? Sometimes expected post-op.

First-degree block? Harmless... until it's not.

But here's the truth: **Bradycardia can be a quiet killer,** and if you don't know what to look for, it can escalate right in front of you. I've seen it happen at the bedside. I've seen it play out in wrongful death cases.

This chapter will teach you how to spot danger early and act fast.

First: When Does "Slow" Become a Problem?

Clinical signs that bradycardia is becoming unstable:

- Altered mental status (confusion, agitation, unresponsiveness)
- Chest pain or pressure
- Hypotension (especially MAP <65)
- Syncope or near-syncope
- Poor cap refill, mottling, cool extremities
- Dizziness or shortness of breath.

Key point:

"Stable bradycardia" isn't about the number; it's about *perfusion.*

If the patient is awake, alert, has a decent pressure, and isn't symptomatic, you may monitor.

But if they're altered, hypotensive, or gray and clammy?

That's not just bradycardia. That's impending cardiac arrest.

Breakdown of Bradycardias and AV Blocks

❖ **Sinus Bradycardia**

- Originates in the SA node, rate < 60 bpm
- Can be normal (athletes, sleep, vagal tone)
- Concerning when: symptomatic, hypotensive, LOC, ischemic

❖ **Junctional Rhythm**

- SA node fails; AV node takes over (rate 40-60 bpm)
- Often, no visible P waves or inverted P waves
- Common post-cardiac surgery, with digoxin toxicity, or ischemia
- Concerning when: **rate is too slow to maintain perfusion,** altered LOC

❖ **First-Degree AV Block**

- PR interval > 0.20 sec, but every P has a QRS
- Usually benign, especially if asymptomatic
- Monitor closely in older adults or with electrolyte issues

- **Second-Degree AV Block Type I (Mobitz I/Wenckebach)**
  - Progressively lengthening PR until a QRS is dropped
  - Usually transient and may resolve
  - Concerning when: **frequent dropped beats,** bradycardia worsens, or symptoms develop

- **Second-Degree AV Block Type II (Mobitz II)**
  - Intermittently dropped QRS with constant PR intervals
  - **More dangerous** - can progress to complete heart block
  - Often requires a pacemaker
  - **Red flag**: Don't ignore "stable" Mobitz II, escalate, monitor closely

- **Third-Degree AV Block (Complete Heart Block)**
  - No relationship between P waves and QRS
  - Atria and ventricles beat independently
  - Rate often 20-40 bpm inadequate for perfusion
  - **Medical emergency** requires pacing and a cardiology consult
  - **Legal danger zone** if not escalated appropriately

When to Escalate Bradycardia

Always escalate when:

- LOC is altered, or the patient is unresponsive
- SBP90 or MAP < 65
- HR < 40 bpm and symptomatic
- Rhythm is junctional, Mobitz II, or 3rd-degree block
- You suspect **hyperkalemia, ischemia**, or **drug overdose**

Call the provider and notify the charge RN. Get a STAT 12-lead. Start oxygen. Prepare to pace.

Lab Link: Hyperkalemia + Bradycardia = Trouble

High potassium can kill silently. The higher it climbs, the slower and wider the rhythm becomes.

This is a common theme in legal cases involving missed bradycardia and cardiac arrest.

Watch for:

- Bradycardia + peaked T waves
- Widened QRS

- Loss of P waves
- Sine wave pattern = pre-arrest

If K > 6 and the HR is < 50, **treat the K and notify fast.**

This is not just lab management; this is a code in slow motion.

Common Causes of Bradycardia Nurses MUST Know

Cause	Why It Matters
Medications	Beta blockers, calcium channel blockers, digoxin, opioids slow SA/AV node conduction
Ischemia	Inferior MI affects RCA → SA/AV node ischemia → bradycardia or blocks
Hyperkalemia	Alters conduction → wide QRS, bradycardia, eventually asystole
Increased ICP	Cushing's triad: bradycardia, hypertension, irregular respirations

Legal Alert: Failure to Escalate = Legal Liability

One of the clearest patterns in nursing malpractice cases is this:

A patient with bradycardia and decreasing LOC was not escalated.

No call made. No 12-lead. No documentation of concern.

The patient coded and died.

In depositions, nurses are asked:

- "Did you recognize this rhythm as dangerous?"
- "Did you document any attempt to notify the provider?"
- "Did you escalate to your charge nurse or call a rapid response?"

In one wrongful death case reviewed, the nurse charted "sinus bradycardia, alert, oriented" at 06:00.

By 07:15, the patient was found unresponsive.

No call. No action. No defense.

If you see a rhythm that doesn't match the patient's status, escalate. Always.

Your license and their life may depend on it.

Nurse Takeaway Checklist

- ✓ Is the patient perfusing? (LOC, BP, skin, UO, etc.)
- ✓ Does the rhythm match the clinical picture?
- ✓ Any red flags for AV block or junctional rhythm?
- ✓ Have I checked labs, especially K and Mg2+?
- ✓ Did I document, notify, and escalate appropriately?

Bradycardia doesn't have to come with fireworks.

Sometimes it's a quiet fade into unconsciousness.

Sometimes it's the *first sign* of something fixable if you catch it early.

If you remember nothing else from this chapter, remember this:

"If the patient looks worse than the monitor, believe the patient."

Next up, we'll look at **tachycardias** and when a fast rhythm means the heart is burning out from the inside.

Chapter 5: Tachycardia Isn't Always a Rhythm Problem

A fast heart isn't always a broken heart, but ignoring why it's fast can be fatal.

The Myth:

"If it's fast, it's a rhythm issue."

The Reality:

Most tachycardias you'll see on a telemetry unit aren't caused by an intrinsic electrical problem. They're **compensatory**—the heart is working overtime because something else is wrong.

Your job is not just to name the rhythm.

Your job is to ask: **What's driving this rate?**

Types of Tachycardia You'll Encounter

❖ **Sinus Tachycardia**

- Originates in the SA node, HR > 100 bpm
- P wave before each QRS, regular rhythm
- **Almost always secondary to something else:**
  - Pain

- Fever
- Anxiety
- Hypovolemia
- Anemia
- Sepsis
- Hypoxia
- PE, tamponade, or other stress states

❖ **Supraventricular Tachycardia (SVT)**

- Rapid rhythm from above the ventricles
- Narrow QRS, often no visible P wave
- Can be triggered by stress, stimulants, or WPW
- Often paroxysmal (starts/stops suddenly)

❖ **Atrial Fibrillation with RVR**

- Chaotic atrial activity with rapid ventricular response
- Irregularly irregular
- Often triggered by infection, fluid shifts, or ischemia
- Rate control vs rhythm control decisions require provider input

❖ **Ventricular Tachycardia**

- Wide complex, HR > 100 bpm
- Can be sustained or nonsustained
- Often due to ischemia, electrolyte issues, or structural disease
- **Medical emergency if sustained and symptomatic**

Ask These Questions Before You Treat a Fast Rhythm

1. Is the patient symptomatic?

- o Chest pain, shortness of breath, dizziness, altered LOC?

2. Is perfusion adequate?

- o BP stable? Skin warm? Urine output okay?

3. Is this rhythm appropriate for the situation?

- o Post-op pain? Fever of 102? Anemia with Hgb 6.8? Sinus tach might be the body's attempt to keep up.

4. Are there reversible causes?

- o Look at oxygenation, fluids, labs, and meds.

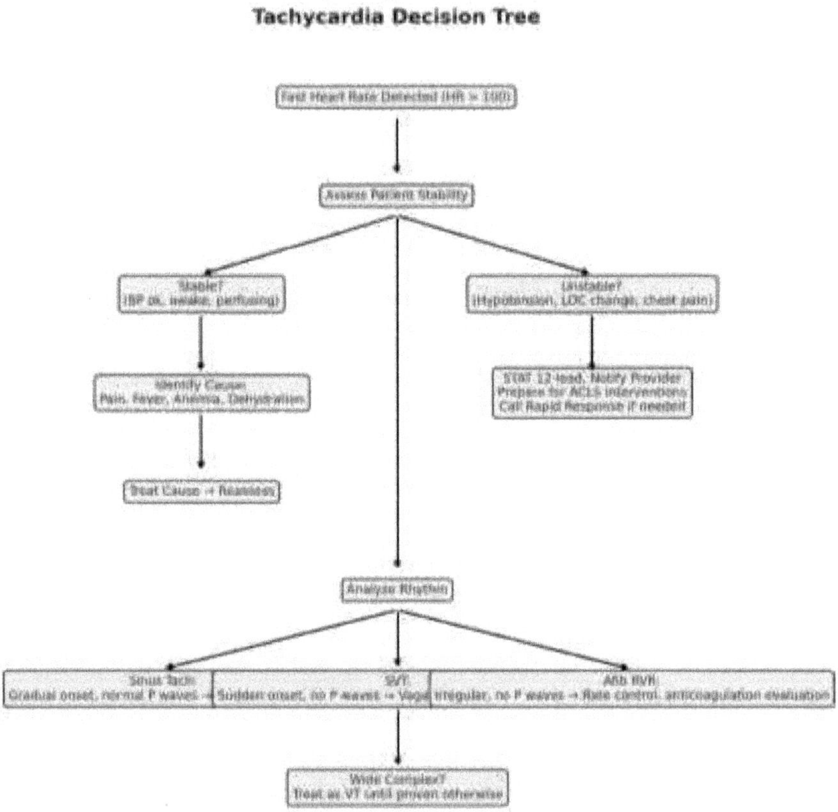

Tachycardia is Often a Symptom, Not the Diagnosis

Treating the rhythm without addressing the cause is like putting a bucket under a leak without fixing the pipe.

Example:

A septic patient is running HR 135 in sinus tachycardia. Giving a beta-blocker might slow the rate, but drop the pressure and kill perfusion.

What they really need: fluids, antibiotics, oxygen, and source control.

When Tachycardia Means Trouble

Tachycardia becomes dangerous when:

- It's **inappropriate** (not explained by a reversible cause)
- It's **sustained and symptomatic** (hypotension, LOC changes)
- It's **ventricular in origin** (VT, Torsades)
- It's worsening despite treatment of the underlying causes

Legal Alert: Don't Miss the Why

In legal reviews, I often see charting like:

"HR 128, sinus tachycardia. Provider aware."

...but no documentation of:

- What caused the tachycardia

- What interventions were done
- How the patient tolerated the rate

Case Example:

A post-op patient remained tachycardic overnight. No fluid bolus was ever given despite low urine output and borderline BP. By morning, they were in hypovolemic shock.

In court, the question was:

"Why was nothing done about this heart rate trend?"

Your documentation should show your thinking:

- *Recognized tachycardia?*
- *Assessed for cause?*
- *Intervened/escalated?*

If it's not in the chart, it didn't happen, and that's where nurses get pulled into legal cases.

Sinus Tachycardia vs SVT vs Afib with RVR

Telemetry will show you a fast rhythm, but what kind of fast rhythm matters?

Rhythm	Key Features on ECG	Clues at the Bedside
Sinus Tachycardia	Normal P before each QRS; HR >100; regular	Often compensatory: fever, anemia, dehydration, hypoxia, pain
Supraventricular Tachycardia (SVT)	Narrow complex; HR 150–250; often no visible P waves	Sudden onset/offset; palpitations, dizziness; often paroxysmal
Atrial Fibrillation with RVR	No discernible P waves; irregularly irregular; HR often 110–160	Often associated with age, infection, post-op, heart disease

Pearl: A gradual speeding up is often sinus tach. A sudden jump from 80 → 180 in one beat? Think SVT.

Compensation vs Decompensation

Sinus Tachycardia is often a *symptom,* not a *disease.*

Your first question: *Is the heart compensating, or is it failing?*

Compensation

- ✓ Warm, awake, oriented
- ✓ BP holding (MAP >= 65)
- ✓ Cause identifiable (fever, pain, hypovolemia)
- ✓ Improving with treatment (fluids, O2, etc.)

Decompensation

- Altered LOC
- Cool, clammy skin
- SBP 90 or MAP 65 despite treatment

- Chest pain, dyspnea, poor urine output
- Rhythm worsening despite interventions

Key action: If you see decompensation signs, **escalate immediately.**

Lab Links That Drive Tachycardia

Trigger	How It Affects the Heart
Anemia (low Hgb/Hct)	Heart speeds up to deliver more oxygen
Dehydration (low preload)	Tachycardia to maintain cardiac output
Infection/Sepsis	Inflammatory response → tachycardia to maintain perfusion
Electrolytes (K^+, Mg^{2+}, Ca^{2+})	Imbalances can trigger ectopy or sustained arrhythmias

Pro tip: Review labs in context. A heart rate of 130 with Hgb 6.0 is compensating. Treat the anemia, not just the rate.

When to Call a Rapid Response

- HR > 130 **and** symptomatic (hypotension, confusion, chest pain)
- New onset tachycardia with **signs of sepsis** (fever, low BP, high lactate)
- Wide-complex tachycardia
- SVT/Afib RVR unresponsive to initial measures
- Sustained rhythm with **declining perfusion** despite

treatment

Document who you notified, what you did, and how the patient responded.

Tachycardia Decision Tree

```
Fast Heart Rate Detected (HR >100) →
│
├► Assess Patient Stability
│        ├─ Stable (BP ok, awake, perfusing)
│        │        ├─ Identify Cause (pain, fever, anemia, dehydration)
│        │        └─ Treat Cause → Reassess
│        │
│        └─ Unstable (hypotension, LOC change, chest pain)
│                 ├─ Get STAT 12-lead, notify provider
│                 ├─ Prepare for ACLS interventions (adenosine, synchronized
cardioversion if indicated)
│                 └─ Call Rapid Response or Code as needed
│
└► Rhythm Analysis
         ├─ Sinus Tach (gradual onset, normal P waves) → Search for cause
         ├─ SVT (sudden onset, no P waves) → Try vagal maneuvers, adenosine
         ├─ Afib RVR (irregular, no P waves) → Rate control, anticoagulation
evaluation
         └─ Wide Complex? → Treat as VT until proven otherwise
```

Case Study: SVT Unresponsive to Vagal – Adenosine Error

Patient:

42-year-old female, post-op day 2 from laparoscopic cholecystectomy. Complains of palpitations, dizzy on standing.

Telemetry:

Narrow-complex tachycardia, HR 180, sudden onset.

Initial Response:

Nurse recognizes likely SVT and attempts vagal maneuvers (cough, bear down), no effect.

BP drops from 118/72 to 92/58. Patient becomes pale, diaphoretic.

Intervention Ordered:

Adenosine 6 mg rapid IV push.

Error Occurs:

Adenosine was given **slowly** over 30 seconds instead of a rapid push followed by a flush.

Result: No effect on rhythm, patient deteriorates further.

Outcome:

Second dose administered correctly, with rapid push rhythm converted to sinus. Patient stabilized.

Legal Learning Point:

- Medication administration for arrhythmias is **high stakes.**
- Adenosine must be pushed **rapidly** through a large bore IV, followed immediately by a flush to reach the heart before

metabolized.

- Delayed or improper administration can prolong instability and lead to worse outcomes.
- Documentation should include the time of rhythm change, interventions attempted, provider notifications, and patient response.

In a deposition, you will be asked:

"Did you follow ACLS guidelines for adenosine administration?"

"Was the medication given per protocol?"

Your documentation is your defense.

Nurse Takeaway Checklist

- ✓ Identify rhythm type (sinus tach, SVT, Afib, RVR)
- ✓ Assess for compensation vs decompensation
- ✓ Check labs: Hgb, electrolytes, infection markers
- ✓ Treat the cause, not just the rate
- ✓ Call the rapid response when unstable
- ✓ Document every step, every notification, every response

Tachycardia isn't always the enemy. Often, it's the body's SOS signal.

Your role: decode the message, treat the cause, and protect the patient from harm.

In the next chapter, we'll dive deeper into **ventricular rhythms** when wide complexes mean the heart is fighting for its life.

Chapter 6: V-Tach, V-Fib, and Torsades -Act Fast, Document Clearly

When a monitor alarm blares and you see wide, chaotic rhythms, seconds matter. These aren't rhythms to "watch." These are **shockable, lethal arrhythmias,** and your ability to recognize, respond, and document can mean the difference between survival and a devastating deposition.

Ventricular Tachycardia (V-Tach)

V-Tach is a **wide-complex rhythm** originating in the ventricles. It can be *monomorphic or polymorphic.*

❖ **Monomorphic V-Tach**

- All QRS complexes look the same.
- Rate often 120-250.
- Usually caused by scar tissue from prior MI, ischemia, or structural disease.
- Can be sustained (lasting >30 sec) or non-sustained.

❖ **Polymorphic V-Tach**

- QRS complexes vary in shape and amplitude.
- Often associated with electrolyte disturbances or prolonged QT.

Key point: Any sustained VT with symptoms (hypotension, altered LOC) is a **medical emergency.**

Ventricular Fibrillation (V-Fib)

- Chaotic, no identifiable QRS complexes.
- Heart is quivering, not pumping.
- No pulse, no perfusion.
- Immediate defibrillation is the only way out.

Torsades de Pointes (a form of polymorphic V-Tach)

"Twisting of the points," the QRS complexes appear to twist around the baseline.

Causes and Triggers:

✓ Low magnesium (hypomagnesemia)

✓ Low potassium (hypokalemia)

- ✓ Prolonged QT interval
- ✓ Certain drugs (see sidebar below)
- ✓ Bradycardia with QT-prolonging drugs

Treatment:

- Magnesium sulfate IV, even if Mg level is normal (stabilizes myocardium)
- Correct K" (target >4.0)
- Overdrive pacing or isoproterenol if recurrent

Lab Links

Abnormal Lab	**Effect on Rhythm**
K <3.5	Promotes ectopy, VT, torsades
Mg < 1.6	Torsades risk ↑, especially with QT-prolonging drugs
Prolonged QTC (>500 ms)	Risk of torsades and sudden death

Sidebar: Common Meds That Prolong QT

Antiarrhythmics: Amiodarone, Sotalol, Procainamide

Antibiotics: Azithromycin, Levofloxacin, Erythromycin

Antipsychotics: Haloperidol, Ziprasidone

Antidepressants: Citalopram, Escitalopram

Others: Methadone, Ondansetron (high doses)

Pro Tip: Review QTc daily in patients on these meds, especially if also hypokalemic or hypomagnesemic.

ACLS in Action

When you see **VT or VF on the monitor:**

1. Check the patient. (Always confirm rhythm with pulse check.)
2. If pulseless, Start CPR and defibrillate ASAP.
3. Follow ACLS algorithm:
    - High-quality CPR minimizes interruptions
    - Shock CPR, Shock Epinephrine, Amiodarone as indicated
    - Treat reversible causes (H's & T's)

Reversible Causes of Cardiac Arrest: The H's and T's

H's	***What It Means***	***Key Interventions***
Hypovolemia	Low circulating volume → PEA or tachycardia	Give IV fluids, blood products
Hypoxia	Low oxygen → brady/asystole/PEA	Ensure airway, ventilation, oxygen delivery
Hydrogen ion (Acidosis)	pH imbalance → arrhythmias	Give sodium bicarb if severe; ventilate
Hypo/Hyperkalemia	Potassium imbalance → VF, VT, asystole	Replace K^+ if low; give calcium, insulin/D50, bicarb if high
Hypothermia	Low body temperature → brady/asystole	Active rewarming measures

T's	***What It Means***	***Key Interventions***
Tension Pneumothorax	Air trapped in pleural space → PEA	Needle decompression, chest tube
Tamponade (Cardiac)	Fluid around heart → PEA	Pericardiocentesis
Toxins	Drug overdose, poisoning	Specific antidotes, decontamination
Thrombosis (Pulmonary)	PE → PEA, sudden collapse	Thrombolytics, embolectomy
Thrombosis (Coronary)	MI → VF, VT, PEA	PCI, thrombolytics

For Torsades:

- Give Magnesium Sulfate 1–2g IV push
- Treat the underlying cause (electrolytes, stop offending meds)

Post-Code Documentation Pitfalls

Clear documentation is your legal armor:

- ✓ Time rhythm was identified, and interventions started.
- ✓ Time of each shock and dose of medications.
- ✓ Patient response after each intervention.
- ✓ Who was notified and when?
- ✓ Any reversible causes addressed?

Legal Alert: In a wrongful death case, attorneys will scrutinize the code record. If times are missing, drugs are undocumented, or rhythm interpretations are unclear, it raises questions about the standard of care.

Nurse Takeaway Checklist

- ✓ Differentiate monomorphic vs polymorphic VT.
- ✓ Recognize torsades and know their triggers.
- ✓ Check electrolytes and QTc in at-risk patients.
- ✓ Act immediately, don't "watch" VT or VF.
- ✓ Document interventions and notifications in real time.

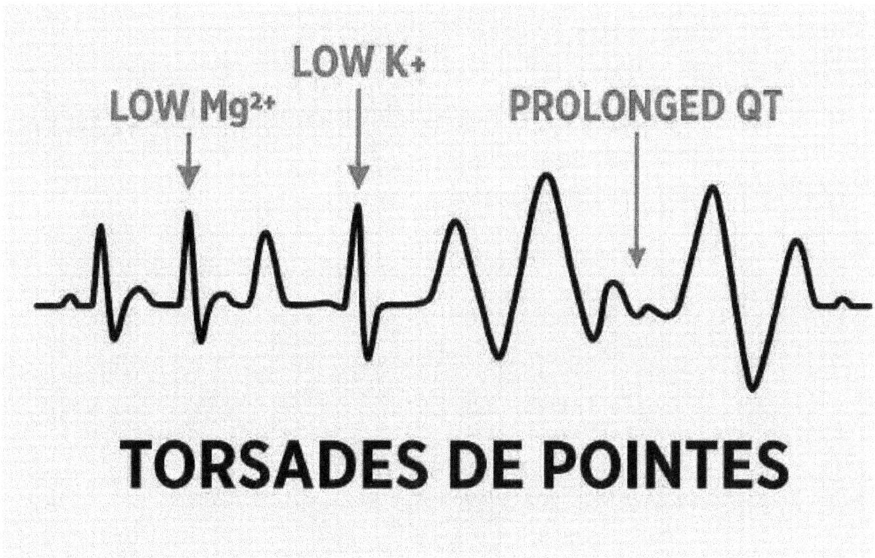

Torsades de pointes with characteristic twisting QRS morphology. Commonly linked to hypomagnesemia, hypokalemia, or QT-prolonging medications.

When the monitor shows VT, VF, or torsades, there is no time for second-guessing.

Act fast, document clearly, and always think about the underlying causes. Your knowledge, speed, and vigilance save lives and protect your license.

Chapter 7: PVCs, PACs, and Ectopy -When to Watch vs. Act

Ectopy happens.

Premature beats are common on any telemetry unit, but the challenge is knowing when they're **benign** and when they're the **canary in the coal mine** warning you of something dangerous brewing.

Understanding Ectopy

Premature Ventricular Complexes (PVCs)

- Wide, bizarre QRS, no preceding P wave.
- Originate in the ventricle before the SA node fires.
- Can occur occasionally in healthy people or signal irritation (ischemia, hypoxia, electrolyte issues).

Premature Atrial Complexes (PACS)

- Early beat with abnormal P wave but narrow QRS.
- Originate in the atria outside the SA node.
- Usually benign but can trigger SVT in susceptible patients.

PVC Patterns to Know

Pattern	What It Looks Like	Significance
Unifocal	All PVCs look the same	Usually from one irritable focus
Multifocal	PVCs look different	Multiple foci → higher risk
Bigeminy	Every other beat is a PVC	May reduce effective cardiac output
Couplets	Two PVCs in a row	Watch closely, could progress
Run of PVCs	≥3 PVCs in a row	*Technically nonsustained VT*
R-on-T Phenomenon	PVC falls on T wave	High risk for VT/VF

Pearl: *An occasional unifocal PVC in a stable patient? Watch Frequent multifocal PVCs in a hypoxic post-op patient? Act.*

Lab Links & Triggers

Trigger	Effect
Low Potassium (K^+)	Ventricular irritability → PVCs, runs
Low Magnesium (Mg^{2+})	Prolonged QT → torsades risk
Hypoxia	Myocardial irritability → ectopy increases
Ischemia	PVC frequency often increases with oxygen demand

Pro Tip:

Always correlate with patient status:

- Are they symptomatic? (palpitations, hypotension, chest pain)
- Are they in a post-op or cardiac context?
- Are labs trending abnormal?

How to Trend and When to Treat

- ✓ Document frequency (occasional, frequent, pattern)
- ✓ Compare to baseline strips
- ✓ Check recent labs (K, Mg, Hgb, O2 saturation)
- ✓ Treat underlying causes:
    - Replace electrolytes (target K^> 4.0, Mg > 2.0)
    - Improve oxygenation
    - Manage ischemia or fluid status

Treatment is needed when:

- PVCs are increasing in frequency or pattern (bigeminy, couplets, runs)
- Associated with hypotension, dizziness, or decreased perfusion
- Occurring in a high-risk setting (post-MI, post-op cardiac)
- R-on-T phenomenon is present

Telemetry Misinterpretation Risks

- PVCs can be over- or under-called by monitors:
    - Motion artifact looks like PVCs but isn't
    - Missing a run of PVCs if alarm parameters aren't set correctly

- Always correlate the monitor strip with the patient's clinical condition and a printed rhythm strip.

Legal Alert

Ignoring frequent PVCs in a post-op patient can lead to disaster.

Case Example:

A post-op cardiac patient was noted to have increasing PVCs on telemetry overnight:

- Bigeminy evolved to couplets and a 4-beat run.
- No labs were checked, no provider notified.
- At 4 AM, patient went into sustained V-Tach cardiac arrest death.

In litigation:

The nurse was asked:

"Why did you not escalate when the frequency of PVCs changed?"

Protect yourself:

- Document the frequency and pattern changes.
- Notify the provider early.
- Record your interventions and patient responses.

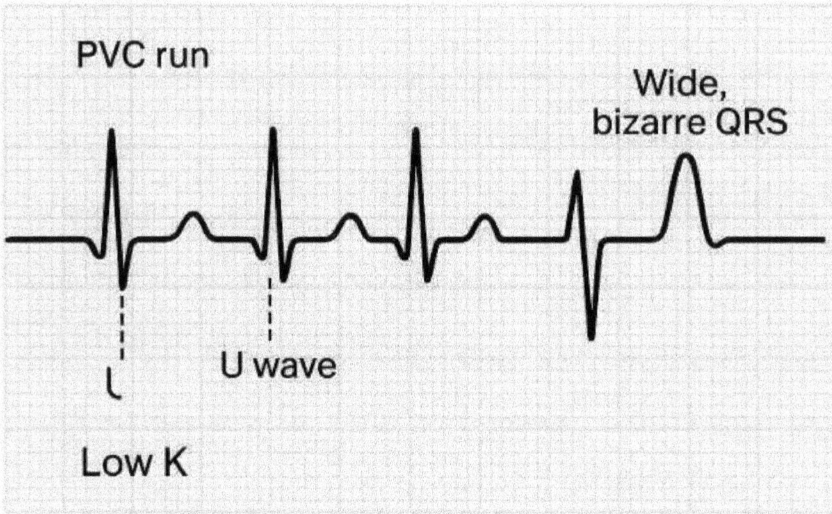

Strip Description:

- Baseline sinus rhythm with intermittent PVCs.
- A clear run of 3 PVCs (nonsustained VT) is highlighted.
- A visible U wave following T waves, indicating low potassium.
- Annotations:
    - "PVC morphology"
    - "Run of PVCs"
    - "U wave (low K")"

Nurse Takeaway Checklist

- ✓ Recognize PVCs vs PACs and patterns (bigeminy, couplets, runs, R-on-T).
- ✓ Correlate ectopy with labs and clinical status.
- ✓ Watch for frequency changes or new patterns.
- ✓ Treat underlying causes early.
- ✓ Document rhythm, frequency, provider notifications, and interventions.

Not all ectopy is dangerous, but **trending changes and acting on them is what protects patients and your license.**

The strip is your starting point. Your critical thinking is what saves lives.

Part 3: Labs + Electrolytes = Rhythm

Chapter 8: Potassium—

Lethal: The Highs, Lows, and Lethal

Potassium is one of the most tightly regulated electrolytes in the body.

Too low, and the heart becomes irritable.

Too high, and the heart can stop cold.

On telemetry, potassium abnormalities write their own story if you know how to read the clues.

The Delicate Balance of K

Normal range: **3.5-5.0 mEq/L**

Even small deviations can lead to significant rhythm changes, especially in vulnerable patients (post-op, renal disease, cardiac history).

Hypokalemia: Low Potassium

Key ECG Findings:

- **U waves** (extra wave after T)
- **Flattened T waves**
- ST depression
- PVCs, runs of VT, torsades risk

Common Causes:

- Diuretics (furosemide, thiazides)
- GI losses (vomiting, diarrhea)
- NG suction
- Excess insulin
- Alkalosis

Treatment Rules:

Replace potassium cautiously:

- **If K** <3.0: IV replacement (typically 10 mEq/hr via peripheral line, up to 20 mEq/hr via central line with monitoring)
- **Always check magnesium first**— low Mg makes K repletion ineffective.
- Reassess labs after replacement.

Hyperkalemia: High Potassium

Key ECG Findings:

- **Peaked T waves** (tall, narrow)
- Prolonged PR interval
- Widened QRS
- **Sine wave pattern**→ impending arrest

Common Causes:

- Renal failure
- Potassium-sparing diuretics (spironolactone)
- ACE inhibitors/ARDS
- Tissue destruction (burns, rhabdomyolysis)
- Hemolysis (false elevation)

Treatment Rules:

Stabilize the myocardium:

- Calcium gluconate or calcium chloride IV
    - ✓ Shift K into cells:
- Insulin + D50
- Albuterol
    - ✓ Remove K from body:
- Furosemide
- Kavexalate

- Dialysis if renal failure

Always Check Magnesium First

Hypomagnesemia often coexists with hypokalemia.

If you replace K without correcting Mg", the potassium will not hold, and arrhythmias can persist.

Rule: Target Mg > 2.0 before or alongside K repletion.

Chart: ECG Changes Based on K+ Levels

K^+ Level	ECG Changes	Clinical Concerns
3.5–5.0 (normal)	Normal P-QRS-T	Stable
3.0–3.4	Flattened T waves, possible U waves	Increased ectopy risk
< 3.0	Prominent U waves, ST depression, PVCs	VT, torsades risk
5.1–5.9	Peaked T waves, normal QRS	Early hyperkalemia
6.0–6.9	Prolonged PR, widened QRS	Progressing hyperkalemia
≥ 7.0	Sine wave pattern	Imminent cardiac arrest

Case Study: Missed Recheck → Cardiac Arrest

Patient:

68-year-old male with end-stage renal disease admitted post-dialysis for pneumonia.

Labs:

Initial K = 6.2mEq / L Calcium given, insulin D50 administered.

Ordered: Recheck potassium in 1 hour.

What Happened:

Recheck was delayed until morning rounds. Overnight telemetry noted a widened QRS and bradycardia.

At 3 AM, the patient developed sine **wave pattern→ asystole.**

Code blue was initiated, but resuscitation was unsuccessful.

Legal Analysis:

- Failure to follow up on critical lab recheck.
- Missed opportunity for dialysis or repeat interventions.
- Documentation gaps: no notes of provider notification when ECG changes were evident.

Protect Yourself:

- Always follow lab-specific recheck orders promptly.
- Document results and actions taken.
- Escalate changes immediately, especially in renal patients.

Nurse Takeaway Checklist

- ✓ Watch telemetry for U waves and flattened T waves in hypokalemia.
- ✓ Peaked T waves and widening QRS in hyperkalemia demand immediate action.
- ✓ Always check magnesium levels first when repleting K
- ✓ Trend labs and document rechecks clearly.
- ✓ Escalate early in renal patients or those with rapid K shifts.

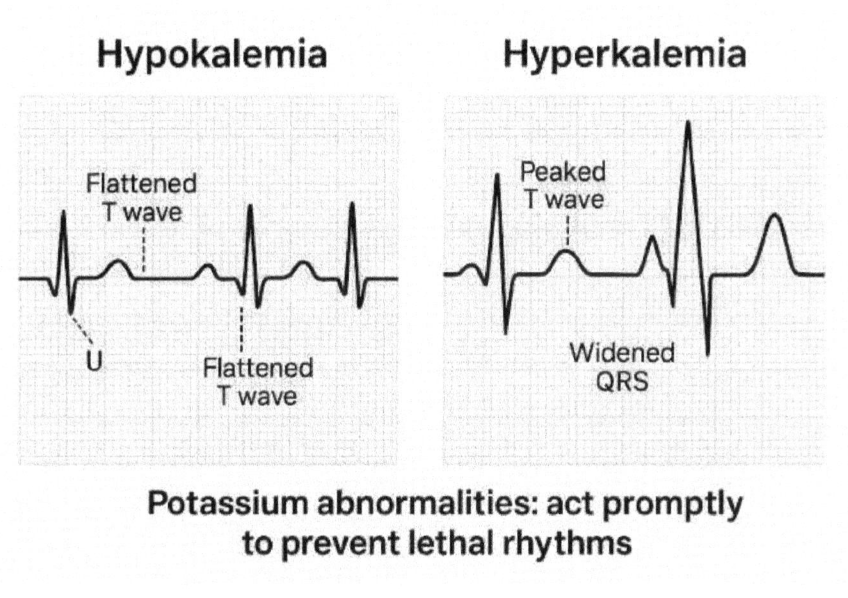

Diagram: Side-by-side strips:

- **Left panel:** Hypokalemia strip with flattened T waves and U waves annotated.
- **Right panel:** Hyperkalemia strip with peaked T waves and

widened QRS annotated.

Below: "Potassium abnormalities: act promptly to prevent lethal rhythms."

Potassium is small but mighty.

It doesn't whisper its warning—it shouts from the ECG.

Your vigilance in trending labs, watching the monitor, and acting quickly will save lives and protect your license.

Chapter 9: Magnesium - The Most Underrated Electrolyte in Nursing

Magnesium doesn't get the spotlight potassium or sodium do, but it is a **quiet powerhouse** in stabilizing cardiac cells.

When magnesium levels drift too low or too high, the heart's rhythm can quickly spiral out of control.

Why Magnesium Matters

Magnesium regulates ion channels, stabilizes myocardial membranes, and works hand-in-hand with potassium.

Without adequate magnesium:

- Potassium replacement won't "stick."
- The myocardium becomes irritable.
- Dangerous rhythms emerge.

Hypomagnesemia (Low Mg^2)

ECG/Telemetry Effects:

- **PVCs** and ventricular ectopy
- **Atrial fibrillation** or atrial flutter
- **Torsades de Pointes** (a form of polymorphic VT)
- Prolonged QT interval

Common Causes:

- Loop and thiazide diuretics
- Alcohol abuse (poor nutrition and increased renal excretion)
- Refeeding syndrome in malnourished patients
- Gl losses (diarrhea, NG suction)

Clinical Pearl:

Magnesium must be replaced before potassium if both are low.

Without adequate magnesium, potassium will simply be wasted by the kidneys.

Replacement Strategy:

- For Mg^{2+} <1.6 mg/dl with arrhythmias: **1-2 grams magnesium sulfate IV over 30-60 min.**
- Monitor for hypotension and respiratory depression with rapid infusion.

Hypermagnesemia (High Mg^{2}")

Less common but dangerous, often seen in:

- Renal failure patients given too much magnesium (antacids, laxatives)
- latrogenic overdose (e.g, OB patients receiving Mg for preeclampsia)

ECG/Telemetry Effects:

- **Bradycardia**
- **Prolonged PR interval**
- **Widened ORS**
- **AV block** or complete heart block in severe cases

Chart: Magnesium Levels and Rhythm Risks

Magnesium Level (mg/dL)	ECG Findings	Clinical Concerns
1.6–2.4 (Normal)	Normal intervals	Stable rhythm
1.2–1.5 (Mild low)	Occasional PVCs, AFib	Monitor trends
< 1.2 (Severe low)	Prolonged QT, Torsades, Polymorphic VT	Replace urgently
> 2.4–4.0 (Mild high)	Slight PR prolongation	Monitor
> 4.0–6.0 (Moderate high)	Bradycardia, AV block	Consider dialysis if renal failure
> 6.0 (Severe high)	Complete heart block, cardiac arrest	Immediate intervention

Legal and Clinical Insight

Magnesium levels are often overlooked in routine telemetry interpretation. But if hypomagnesemia goes uncorrected, the resulting torsades or refractory hypokalemia can be catastrophic--and **chart reviews will ask why no replacement was given.**

Nurse Takeaway Checklist

- ✓ Always check magnesium with potassium abnormalities.
- ✓ Replace Mg before K" for lasting effect.
- ✓ Watch for PVCs, AFib, torsades in low Mg
- ✓ Monitor for bradycardia and blocks in high Mg",
- ✓ Document replacement, lab trends, and provider communication.

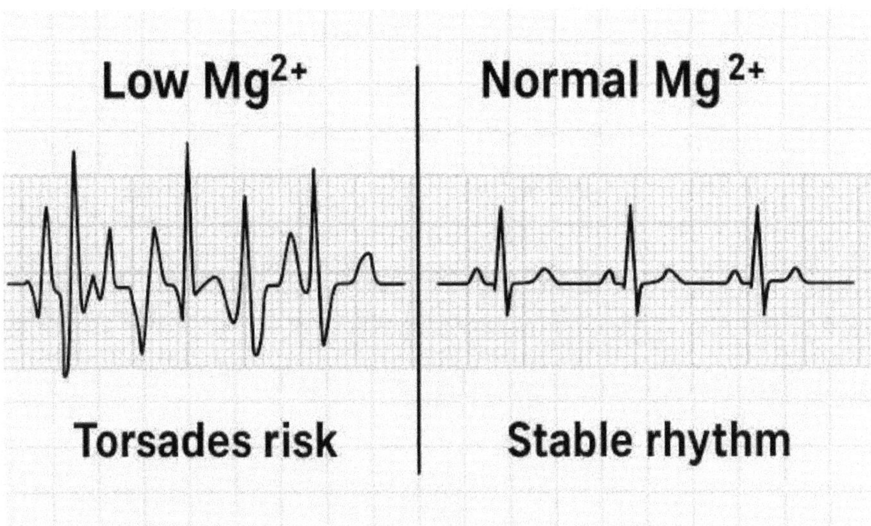

A side-by-side comparison of ECG strips:

- **Left Panel (Low Mg"):** Shows PVCs and prolonged QT with an annotation "Torsades risk."
- **Right Panel (Normal Mg"):** Shows a stable sinus rhythm

with normal intervals, annotated "Normal Mg","

- **"Magnesium Levels and Rhythms: Low Mg^{2+} →Ectopy and torsades risk. Normal Mg^{2+} →Stable rhythm."**

Magnesium may be underrated, but as a telemetry nurse or legal nurse consultant, you know better:

Magnesium is the rhythm stabilizer. Treat it with the same urgency as potassium, your patient's heart depends on it.

Chapter 10: Calcium, Sodium, and ABG Clues You Can't Miss

In cardiac monitoring, it's easy to focus only on potassium and magnesium.

But calcium, sodium, and even your ABG results carry critical clues about rhythm changes and neurologic instability. Missing these can cost precious time, and in a legal review, those missed clues become red flags.

Calcium: More Than Bones

Calcium plays a key role in cardiac conduction and muscle contraction.

Too low or too high, and the heart's electrical system reacts.

Low Calcium (Hypocalcemia)

ECG Findings:

- **Prolonged QT interval**
- May progress to torsades or other ventricular dysrhythmias
- Often seen in renal disease, massive transfusions, or low albumin states

Clinical Signs:

- Muscle twitching
- Numbness/tingling around the mouth
- **Chvostek's sign** (facial twitch with cheek tap)

Pro Tip:

Always use a **corrected QT calculator** when calcium is low.

Low albumin can falsely lower total calcium, but the *ionized calcium* is what truly matters.

High Calcium (Hypercalcemia)

ECG Findings:

- Shortened QT interval
- Risk of arrhythmias with very high levels

Clinical Signs:

- Lethargy, weakness
- Renal stones, confusion

Sodium: The Neuro-Cardiac Connection

Sodium abnormalities are often underestimated in telemetry patients, but they dramatically affect the brain and, secondarily, the heart.

Hyponatremia

- **Altered LOC, confusion, seizures**
- Can lead to secondary hypoxia and arrhythmias if seizures occur

Hypernatremia

- Neurologic irritability, restlessness
- Risk of dehydration and hypovolemia, tachycardia, hypotension

Pearl: *Any rhythm change with unexplained altered LOC should prompt a sodium check.*

ABGS: What Acidosis Does to the Heart

Acidosis (pH < 7.35):

- Myocardium becomes irritable
- Decreased contractility→ hypotension
- Potassium shifts **out of cells**→ rising serum K^+ →peaked T

waves, widened QRS, and potential VF/VT

Alkalosis (pH > 7.45):

- Potassium shifts **into cells**→ low serum K^+→ U waves, ectopy
- Coronary vasoconstriction→ ischemic changes

Metabolic Clues in Rhythm Changes

- **Lactate rising?** Look for sepsis-induced acidosis→ K shifts arrhythmias.
- **Bicarbonate low?** Acidosis is likely driving QT prolongation or ventricular irritability.
- **Rapid pH swings?** Watch telemetry closely for ectopy or conduction changes.

Sidebar: How Acidosis Affects K Levels and Rhythms

Acidosis drives potassium **out of cells** →serum K^+ rises.

On ECG: **peaked T waves, wide QRS, bradycardia, or VF risk.**

Correcting pH often improves potassium levels and rhythm stability.

Quick Tip

Use a corrected QT calculator when calcium is low.

- Hypocalcemia prolongs the QT, but low albumin can make total calcium appear low when ionized calcium is normal.
- Before treating or alarming providers, double-check with the corrected value or ionized calcium level.

Nurse Takeaway Checklist

- ✓ Check QT intervals in low calcium states, watch for twitching, and Chvostek's sign.
- ✓ Track sodium trends in patients with altered LOC or seizure activity.
- ✓ Review ABGs for acidosis/alkalosis driving rhythm changes.
- ✓ Remember metabolic shifts (K". Mg) are interconnected.
- ✓ Document lab reviews, provider notifications, and interventions clearly.

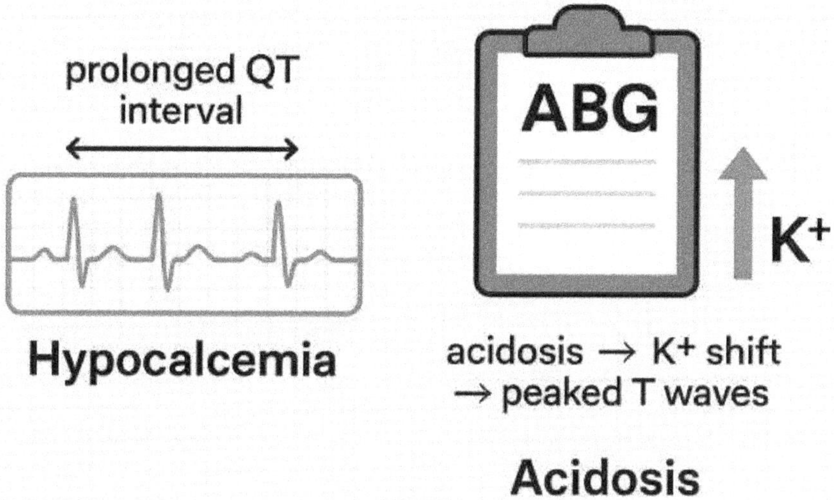

Electrolyte and ABG Clues in Rhythm Interpretation

- Left: ECG strip with **prolonged QT** and an annotation: *Hypocalcemia.*
- Right: ABG panel icon with arrows showing acidosis→ K^+ shift →peaked T *waves*.

Calcium, sodium, and ABGs are often hidden in plain sight. Your vigilance in correlating these values with rhythm changes can prevent seizures, arrests, and lawsuits. **Read beyond the strip—read the labs.**

Part 4: Legal Nursing Wisdom

Chapter 11: Documentation That Protects You (and Your Patient)

When a cardiac rhythm goes wrong, your words on the chart become just as important as your actions at the bedside.

Defense attorneys, risk managers, and expert witnesses comb through your notes line by line. What they find—or don't find—can determine the outcome of a lawsuit.

This chapter gives you practical strategies to document clearly, objectively, and legally sound in any rhythm-related situation.

What Defense Attorneys Look for in Your Note

- **Timeline clarity:**
  When did you notice the change? When did you act?
  Time stamps matter.
- **Escalation evidence:**
  Who did you notify, when, and what was their response?
  Did you go up the chain if the patient worsened?
- **Orders followed (or not followed):**
  Did you carry out the orders promptly? If not, why not?

Document barriers, refusals, or contraindications.

- **Clinical reasoning**:

  Your note should show you recognized the problem and acted within your scope.

- **Objective tone:**

  Avoid emotional wording or blame. Stick to the facts.

Write Objective, Not Emotional Notes

- Risky:

"Patient was crashing, and no one would help. I begged the MD to come see them."

- Safe:

"At 0215, telemetry showed sustained VT. Patient pale, diaphoretic, BP 80/40. MD Johnson notified at 0218; awaiting orders. Rapid Response was activated at 0220."

Tip: Replace subjective feelings with observable signs and actions.

Saying "MD aware" Isn't Enough

A vague note like *"MD aware"* leaves too many unanswered questions in court:

- **Which MD?**
- **When were they notified?**
- **What did they say or order?**
- **What did you do in response?**

Example Upgrade:

Instead of: "MD aware.

Write: "0218: Dr. Patel notified of frequent PVCs with a run of 3 beats. Ordered K^+ replacement and repeat BMP at 0600. K^+ 3.0→40 mEq KCI PO given at 0225."

Before/After: Real vs. Risky Documentation

Risky Note	Improved Note
"Patient having weird beats. Will monitor."	"Telemetry showing frequent PVCs (approx. 6/min). Patient denies chest pain or SOB. K^+ 3.1. Dr. Smith notified at 1800; order received for 40 mEq KCl IV over 4 hrs. Infusion started 1815. Will recheck labs at 2200."
"Patient got worse, MD aware."	"0030: Telemetry change to 2nd degree Type II block. HR 38, BP 84/52. Dr. Lee notified 0033; atropine 0.5 mg IV given at 0035 per order. External pacing pads applied at 0037."
"Rapid Response called. Hope they get here soon."	"0715: Rapid Response Team called for symptomatic bradycardia (HR 30, BP 70/40). Team arrived 0718. Transcutaneous pacing initiated. Patient transferred to ICU at 0730 with continuous monitor."

Checklist: What to Include in a Rhythm-Related Progress Note

- **Time stamps:** exact times of changes, notifications, and interventions.
- **Rhythm description:** what you see on telemetry (PVCs, blocks, runs of VT).
- **Patient response:** symptoms, vitals, LOC.
- **Actions taken:** oxygen applied, pads placed, meds given.
- **Provider notifications:** name, time, orders received.
- **Escalation steps:** Rapid Response, charge RN, ICU transfer.
- **Follow-up:** repeat labs, reassess vitals, and rhythm changes after intervention.

Clear, factual documentation protects your patient's safety and **your license**. In court, your note is your voice when you're not in the room to explain yourself.

Write every entry as if someone will read it aloud in front of a jury one day—because they might.

Chapter 12: Alarm Fatigue, Monitoring Errors, and Missed Deterioration

Telemetry saves lives--but only if we hear what it's saying.

In today's high-acuity environments, constant alarms can blend into background noise, leads can be misplaced, and critical information can fall through the cracks during handoff. These lapses are not just clinical errors; they can create devastating legal exposure.

Alarm Fatigue: A Growing Threat

Alarm fatigue happens when staff become desensitized to frequent, non-actionable alarms. But when a truly dangerous rhythm occurs and no one responds, the consequences are dire.

Real Risk:

When alarms are muted, silenced, or limits are widened without a proper rationale and documentation, **liability falls on the team and individual caregivers.**

Key Question in Court:

"Why was the alarm disabled?"

If you can't show a valid, documented clinical reason, your actions may be viewed as negligence.

Alarms Turned Off-Who's Liable?

- The **primary nurse** is responsible for ensuring alarms are active and set to appropriate parameters.
- If you delegate monitoring to another staff member (telemetry tech or float nurse), **you retain accountability** for the patient's response unless a formal handoff occurs.
- Hospitals have policies: failure to follow them (e.g., leaving a monitor in "standby" mode) can trigger **med-mal claims against both the nurse and facility.**

Delegation vs. Abandonment

Delegation:

- Assigning a qualified individual a task within their scope while maintaining oversight.

Abandonment:

- Failing to monitor or respond to patient needs after accepting responsibility.

Example:

- Delegating rhythm review to a telemetry technician is acceptable.
- Leaving a high-risk patient unmonitored during transport or

turning off alarms for convenience? That's abandonment.

Missed Arrhythmia Alerts - Med-Mal Triggers

- **Common causes:**
    - Alarm thresholds set incorrectly
    - Leads disconnected and not reattached
    - Ignoring frequent PVCs or runs of VT
- **Legal scrutiny:**
    - Documentation gaps ("no note of alarm settings")
    - Lack of timely response despite monitor evidence

Handoff Failures with Unstable Rhythms

"Handoff is a transfer of responsibility, not just information."

When one nurse reports off and another takes over, every critical rhythm detail must transfer.

Missed Details →Missed treatment→ bad outcomes→ lawsuits.

Key elements to report:

- Current rhythm and any recent changes

- Electrolyte trends
- Recent interventions and pending orders
- Alarm parameters and any adjustments made

Case Study: Missed Lead Placement Error → Delayed MI Diagnosis

Patient:

A 54-year-old male was admitted for chest pain. The telemetry strip showed nonspecific changes. Leads were applied incorrectly (RA/LA reversed).

What Happened:

- ST elevations were masked by lead misplacement.
- Alarms repeatedly noted "lead fail," but staff silenced alarms due to "artifact."
- No provider escalation occurred despite ongoing symptoms.

Outcome:

- Patient's MI was diagnosed 8 hours later after deterioration and troponin rise.
- Family sued for failure to monitor and a delay in diagnosis.

Legal Review Focused On:

- Alarm settings (muted without documentation)
- Lack of documentation of lead checks
- No notation of provider notification despite ongoing symptoms

Legal Alert: When Nurse-to-Nurse Handoff Becomes a Lawsuit

In litigation, attorneys often ask:

"Was this information handed off?"

"Did the receiving nurse know the patient was unstable?"

If critical rhythm changes or concerns are not communicated, both nurses can face scrutiny.

A written or electronic handoff tool is only as good as what you put in it:

- If you omit "frequent runs of VT overnight," you've set the next nurse up for failure-and yourself for legal exposure.

Nurse Takeaway Checklist

- Never mute or disable alarms without a documented clinical rationale.
- Confirm lead placement on admission, after procedures, and if alarms persist.
- Respond to and document every significant arrhythmia alert.
- During handoff, clearly communicate rhythm changes, interventions, and pending concerns.
- Remember: **Delegation does not remove your responsibility.**

Alarm fatigue is real, but so is your responsibility

Your notes, your handoffs, and your vigilance are your best defense. When you hear that alarm, ask yourself:

If this went to court, could I prove I responded appropriately?

Chapter 13: When to Escalate and How to Cover Yourself

Escalation is one of the most powerful tools you have to save a life and protect your license.

But many nurses hesitate, worried they'll seem insubordinate or overreacting.

In reality, failing to escalate can be far more dangerous both clinically and legally.

Advocacy vs. Insubordination

Advocacy:

- Speaking up for the patient when their condition worsens or orders are delayed.
- Using clinical data (vitals, rhythm, labs) to justify your concerns.
- Following the facility policy to notify providers or activate rapid response.

Insubordination:

- Refusing reasonable orders without a documented clinical reason.
- Ignoring the chain of command and going rogue without evidence.

Bottom Line: Advocacy is not insubordination when you are acting on behalf of patient safety. In a deposition, the question will be:

"Did you do everything reasonable to escalate the situation?"

Chain of Command

Hospitals have a clear chain of command-know yours:

1. **Primary Provider (MD/APP)** → notify first.
2. **Charge Nurse/Supervisor** → if no response or disagreement.
3. **Department Director/House Supervisor** → escalate if concern unresolved.
4. **Rapid Response or Code Team** → if patient unstable or deteriorating.

Document each step with **times, names, and responses.**

SBAR That Protects You Legally

Using SBAR (Situation, Background, Assessment, Recommendation) is not just good practice—**it creates a record of clear, concise advocacy.**

Example:

S: "Dr. Patel, this is RN Smith on 3B. I'm calling about Mr. Jones, his heart rate is 38 with 2nd-degree AV block."

B: "He was admitted with pneumonia, on beta-blocker therapy. No prior history of bradycardia."

A: "Telemetry shows worsening block; BP 84/50, patient diaphoretic."

R: "I recommend evaluation now and orders for atropine or pacing pads. Should I call Rapid Response?"

✓ This structure shows you recognized the issue, gathered data, and made a recommendation.

Refusal to Act or Document = Shared Liability

If you see a rhythm change, a critical lab, or a patient deteriorating and do nothing or fail to document your actions, you may share liability with the primary team.

Remember:

- "I didn't think it was important" does not stand up in court.
- "I told someone verbally" is not enough without documentation.

Flowchart: When to Escalate Rhythm/Lab Concerns

```
              Monitor or Lab Abnormality Detected
                              ↓
             Assess Patient (vitals, symptoms, LOC)
                              ↓
Is patient unstable? (SBP<90, HR<40 or >130, new chest pain, AMS)
                   ┌──────────┴──────────────┐
            | YES (unstable)          | NO (stable)
                   |                         |
       Rapid Response & Notify MD    Notify MD with SBAR
     Apply emergency interventions  Document call & response
                   ↓                         ↓
          If no response, escalate up chain of command
                              ↓
      Document all calls, times, names, and actions taken
```

Template: Escalation Note Language for Self-Protection

Time-stamped, factual, and clear.

Safe Note Example:

2135: Telemetry showed a new onset of 2nd degree AV block. HR 38, BP 84/50, patient diaphoretic and dizzy. Dr. Patel notified at 2138 via SBAR; recommended atropine/pacing evaluation. No new orders at this time. Charge nurse informed at 2140. Rapid Response was activated at 2142 due to continued instability. Patient transferred to ICU at 2200.

Risky Note Example:

Patient not doing well, MD aware.

Nurse Takeaway Checklist

- ✓ Know your chain of command and follow it step by step.
- ✓ Advocate for patient safety-advocacy is not insubordination.
- ✓ Use SBAR to communicate and protect yourself legally.
- ✓ Document every escalation: time, name, action, and outcome.
- ✓ Never rely on vague statements; clarity is your defense.

Escalation isn't about creating conflict, it's about preventing tragedy.

If a rhythm or lab concerns you enough to hesitate, it's serious enough to **document and escalate.**

Your future self (and your patient) will thank you.

Part 5: Nursing with Eyes Wide Open

Chapter 14: Pattern Recognition = Nurse Intelligence

Nurses are more than task doers; we are pattern recognizers.

Telemetry isn't just about seeing a strip; it's about connecting **rhythms, vitals, and labs** into a story before anyone else does. That's real nurse intelligence and—it's what saves lives.

Why We Don't Just "Follow Orders"

Following orders is not enough when the patient is actively deteriorating.

Your license, your assessment skills, and your ability to see patterns make you the first line of defense.

Orders are reactive. **Pattern recognition is proactive.**

Legal Insight:

In court, attorneys often ask: *"Was there evidence the patient was deteriorating before the event?"* If those signs were on the monitor or in the chart and nobody acted, liability follows.

Pre-Code Patterns Nurses Miss

Here are red flags that often show up hours before a code event:

- **Telemetry:** Frequent PVCs, short runs of VT, or new bundle branch blocks
- **Vitals:** Rising heart rate with falling BP, or persistent mild hypotension
- **Labs:** K dropping to 3.0 with rising creatinine; magnesium trending down
- **Neuro:** Subtle confusion, restlessness, or anxiety
- **Output:** Decreasing urine output despite stable IV fluids

These aren't isolated data points—they're patterns.

How Vitals + Labs + Rhythm Tell a Story

Example 1:

- HR climbing from 90→110→125 over 4 hours.
- Temp 101.4→102.1. BP trending down, lactate rising
- Rhythm: sinus tachycardia.

✓ *The story:* Sepsis is brewing. Call the provider, escalate.

Example 2:

- PVCs increasing per hour, K^+ 3.2, Mg^{2+} 1.4

✓ *The story:* Electrolyte instability→treat before torsades occur.

Recognizing Sick vs. Stable

Stable:

- Rhythm irregularities with no symptoms, good BP, good perfusion.

Sick:

- Rhythm changes with symptoms: hypotension, altered LOC, chest pain, diaphoretic, cool extremities.

When in doubt, err on the side of "sick" until proven otherwise.

Case Study: "The Patient Looked Fine..." But Wasn't

Patient:

65-year-old female post-op, on telemetry. Vitals within normal limits, but HR gradually increased from 88→115 over 6 hours. The telemetry tech noted occasional PVCs. K that morning: 3.1. No interventions ordered.

What Happened:

- At 0200, the patient suddenly developed torsades and coded.
- Review showed a pattern of increasing ectopy, trending tachycardia, and **hypokalemia** that was never escalated.

Key Takeaway:

She "looked fine" until she wasn't. A nurse who connected the dots could have triggered electrolyte replacement and a different outcome.

Sidebar: How Nurses Save Lives Before Doctors Know There's a Problem

Doctors rely on your assessments. They aren't at the bedside every hour you are. Your pattern recognition often detects deterioration before labs come back or before the provider rounds.

Examples:

- Recognizing a widening QRS on telemetry before hyperkalemia is confirmed.
- Noticing a trend of falling urine output with rising HR before sepsis criteria are met.
- Catching subtle changes in mental status before neuro decline becomes irreversible.

Your vigilance and communication bridge the gap between data and action.

Nurse Takeaway Checklist

- Don't just record data—**connect it.**
- Look for trends, not just isolated numbers.
- Treat sinus tachycardia as a symptom, not a rhythm problem, until proven otherwise.
- Document and escalate patterns, not just single events.
- Trust your gut—if it feels "off," dig deeper.

Pattern recognition is not extra work—it's core to what makes nursing a profession.

You are not "just following orders."

You are actively interpreting and intervening long before a provider arrives. That's how nurses save lives and protect themselves in the process.

Chapter 15: From Task-Based to Thinking Nurse

Many nurses begin their careers in survival mode, checking tasks off a list, documenting, and hoping they don't miss anything. But safe cardiac monitoring requires more than task completion.

It requires **critical thinking, pattern recognition, and the courage to speak up.**

This chapter is about making that shift and helping others do the same.

Building Confidence Through Clinical Questions

A thinking nurse asks why. Not to challenge, but to learn and to connect the dots.

- **Instead of:** "The doctor ordered potassium."
- **Ask:** "Why is potassium being replaced? What rhythm changes am I watching for?"
- **Instead of:** "Telemetry shows PVCs."
- **Ask:** "What could be causing ectopy in this patient? Labs? Ischemia? Meds?"

The more you ask, the more confident you become and the more you anticipate problems before they escalate.

Preempting with Purpose

Preempting isn't guessing—it's anticipating.

When you see early warning signs and act before deterioration:

- You prevent rapid responses.
- You prevent legal exposure.
- You build trust with your team and providers.

Example:

You see K trending low (3.2) and PVCs increasing. You don't wait for a code. You call for replacement, document the conversation, and stop the rhythm storm before it starts.

Helping New Grads Understand the "Why" Behind Interventions

New graduates often focus on "what" they have to do, not "why" they are doing it.

Teach them:

- What different electrolytes do to cardiac conduction?
- Why a patient with PVCs might need magnesium before potassium.
- How an early rhythm change could signal sepsis or hypoxia.

When they understand the why, they stop blindly following orders and start **thinking like nurses.**

Creating a Culture of Accountability

Thinking nurses foster accountability:

- We share trends and concerns openly.
- We encourage escalation without fear of "bothering" someone.
- We document clearly and thoroughly because we know our notes protect patients—and us.

Culture starts with one nurse modeling the behavior.

Reflection: A Personal Story

Years ago, I was monitoring a post-op cardiac patient. His vitals were within normal limits, but I noticed his telemetry showed short runs of ventricular bigeminy. His potassium that morning was 3.3.

Something in my gut said this wasn't right. I called the resident, explained the pattern, and requested labs and replacement. He sighed but ordered it. Two hours later, the patient's labs came back: potassium had dropped to 2.9. We replaced aggressively, and those runs stopped. Later, the resident thanked me for catching it early. That moment reminded me that speaking up matters, even when no one else sees what you see.

Worksheet: What to Teach New Grads About Telemetry and Labs

Instructions: Use this worksheet as a teaching tool during precepting or orientation.

Topic	Key Points to Teach	Example or Practice Question
Basic ECG Interpretation	Identify P, QRS, T; normal intervals	"Show me a strip and tell me what you see."
Common Rhythms	Sinus rhythms, PVCs, blocks, tachyarrhythmias	"What's the difference between sinus tachycardia and SVT?"
Electrolyte Links	K^+ = T waves; Mg^{2+} = PVCs/Torsades; Ca^{2+} = QT interval	"What lab would you check for frequent PVCs?"
Symptom Correlation	Don't just read a strip—look at vitals and patient	"If the HR is 45 but BP is stable, what next?"
Escalation Pathways	Chain of command, SBAR	"How would you call the MD about this strip?"
Documentation	Objective, time-stamped notes	"Write a note for a run of VT with intervention."

Reflection Question for New Grads:

- *What patterns have you noticed that made you speak up?*

- *If you see something concerning, who do you call first?*
- *How will you document to show you acted on what you saw?*

Nurse Takeaway Checklist

- ✓ Ask clinical questions and dig deeper than tasks.
- ✓ Teach the "why" behind interventions to new nurses.
- ✓ Create a culture of escalation and accountability.
- ✓ Remember: *Your vigilance is what saves lives before a provider ever knows there's a problem.*

Becoming a thinking nurse isn't about experience alone—it's about curiosity, advocacy, and courage. Every shift is an opportunity to grow that mindset and teach it to others. And in doing so, you protect patients, your team, and your own professional integrity.

Conclusion: Your Monitor Can Save a Life—But Only If You Read It Right

A monitor is only as powerful as the nurse interpreting it.

It can alarm, display, and trend all day long—but it does **not** think. **You do.**

Your vigilance, the way you correlate rhythm changes with labs, vitals, and patient symptoms, is what turns data into action. It's what prevents codes, protects patients, and safeguards your license.

Your Monitor Is a Tool, not a Brain

- The screen shows you patterns.
- **You decide what those patterns mean.**
- Your critical thinking transforms a beep into a life-saving intervention.

Your Vigilance Matters

Every time you:

- Notice a subtle rhythm change,
- Catch a potassium trending down,

- Escalate a concern before deterioration,
- ...you are practicing at the highest level of nursing intelligence.

Final Encouragement

Stay curious.

Ask *why* every day.

Think critically, connect the dots, and never stop learning.

Document as if every word could be read in court, because it might.

Your eyes on that monitor, your brain interpreting it, and your charting that tells the story—these are what keep patients alive and keep you protected.

You've got this.

Keep learning.

Keep thinking.

And remember:

Your monitor can save a life—

but only if you read it right.

Your monitor can save a life—

but only if you know how to read it.

In *What Every Nurse Must See Before a Code: Telemetry Secrets,* veteran cardiac nurse and legal nurse consultant Kristina Michelle, BSN, RN, pulls back the curtain on telemetry interpretation and clinical decision-making. More than just waveforms on a screen, these patterns tell a story—and the nurse at the bedside is the first to read it.

With clarity, case studies, and easy-to-follow visuals, Kristina teaches you how to:

- ✓ Recognize pre-code patterns most nurses miss
- ✓ Correlate rhythms with labs, vitals, and symptoms
- ✓ Intervene early before compensation turns to collapse
- ✓ Document in ways that protect both your patient and your license

From bradycardias to torsades, from potassium pitfalls to magnesium mysteries, you'll learn not only what you're seeing on the monitor but *why it matters*—and how to act on it.

Stay curious. Think critically. Chart like it counts—because it does.

Whether you're a new grad hungry for a deeper understanding or a seasoned nurse looking to sharpen your edge, this book will help you save lives, build confidence, and protect your practice every shift.

About the Author

Kristina Michelle, BSN, RN, is a veteran cardiac nurse with over 27 years of experience in telemetry, progressive care, and critical care settings. She has spent her career interpreting complex rhythms, correlating labs with patient symptoms, and mentoring nurses to build confidence at the bedside. Kristina is passionate about teaching others how to think beyond tasks, recognize subtle patterns before deterioration, and document in ways that protect both patients and their licenses. When she's not writing or teaching, she enjoys sharing her knowledge with new generations of nurses and inspiring them to see the art and science of nursing in every rhythm strip.

www.ingramcontent.com/pod-product-compliance
Lightning Source LLC
La Vergne TN
LVHW050921210926
848482LV00012B/488